Increase Your Peace from A to Z

Simple Steps to Find Calm Amid Chaos

Lea Grimaldi

Copyright © 2019 Lea Grimaldi

ISBN: 978-1-64438-872-3

Published by BookLocker.com, Inc., St. Petersburg, Florida.

Library of Congress Cataloging in Publication Data
Grimaldi, Lea
Increase Your Peace from A to Z: Simple Steps to Find Calm Amid Chaos by Lea Grimaldi
Body, Mind and Spirit | Health and Fitness | Self-help
Library of Congress Control Number: 2019943773

Printed on acid-free paper.

Booklocker.com, Inc.
2019

First Edition

Table of Contents

How to Use This Book

This book is intended for anyone who feels anxious, overwhelmed, or stressed out and doesn't know where to turn. It is an easy, quick read with guidelines on how you can increase your peace and find calm every day. Think of it as a mini-directory for stress relief. You may want to read the entire book and then use it as one tool in your toolbox to help you deal with stressful moments. I experience occasional anxiety and have often wished for something like this book when I need to talk myself down from the ledge.

If you are experiencing an especially stressful moment, it is my hope that you can open the book and quickly find a way to calm down. If you only have five or ten minutes, turn to B and do some quick breathing exercises. Even taking one mindful, conscious, deep breath will immediately make you feel better, and you'll start to calm down. If you have more time, you can turn to C and call a friend.

I know how debilitating and life interrupting anxiety and panic attacks can be. It is my mission to provide simple, inexpensive, and practical solutions to try right now. Here's to happier, healthier days and peaceful nights. xo

Chapter 1

A: Affirmations

"An affirmation opens the door, it's a beginning point on the path to change." Louise L. Hay

An affirmation is a positive statement focusing on something we want to manifest. I have been using affirmations to improve my life since first being introduced to them many years ago. The key with affirmations is to put them in your own words and state them in the present tense, as if what you seek is already real. For example, if you are having difficulty with a relationship, state the affirmation as though the relationship is exactly as you would like it to be.

How to practice: It is a good idea to say your affirmations in the morning, to set the tone for the day. I like to do ten sets of ten, for a total of one hundred. If you are feeling rushed and stressed, start with this:

I am calm. There is plenty of time for me to achieve all that I need to achieve today.

Below are some specific examples by category.

HEALTH

If you are embarking on a lifestyle change such as improved fitness and diet, target your affirmations to that area. These can also apply if you have a chronic illness or condition.

- *I enjoy perfect health. I have plenty of energy to accomplish what I want to do. I eat healthy foods that nourish my body and I drink enough water to stay hydrated.*
- *My body is strong and getting stronger each day. I enjoy exercise for how it makes me feel.*
- *I always have plenty of energy to do everything I want to do.*
- *I love my body.*

- ◆ *I am healthy and happy in mind, body, and spirit.*

LOVE

SELF-LOVE

Self-love is the most important type of love, so start here.

- ◆ *I love and accept myself completely.*
- ◆ *I am worthy of love and joy.*
- ◆ *I take the time to look after myself.*

ROMANTIC LOVE

- ◆ *I attract the perfect partner into my life.*
- ◆ *My partner loves me and I love them. They are kind, smart, funny, and treat me well.*
- ◆ *I have a great partner. We have fun together and want the same things out of life.*

FAMILIAL LOVE

If the area that needs work is your relationship with your family of origin or a specific person, make the affirmation specific too.

- *My relationship with my father is great. He supports me and I enjoy spending time with him.*
- *I love my family and have a good relationship with them. I am thankful to have them in my life.*
- *My sister and I enjoy a close and loving relationship.*

GENERAL LOVE (Friends, Coworkers, Life)

- *My relationships are full of love and positive connections.*
- *I have self-love, friend love, family love, and romantic love in my life.*
- *I am content with my life and things work out for me.*

ABUNDANCE

- *I graciously and freely accept the abundance that surrounds me, and I know that I deserve the best in everything I do. I accept this abundance into my open heart and make it mine.*
- *I accept and receive all the good that is coming to me.*

MONEY

- *Money flows to me. I am a money magnet.*
- *I have all the money I need to live happily. I easily make more than enough money to take care of my needs.*

WORK

- *I have a job that I love. I do fulfilling work with people I respect and enjoy.*
- *I am always getting new opportunities to make money doing work that fulfills me.*

♦ *My job doesn't feel like work, because it brings me joy.*

LACK OF TIME

If you feel stressed and overwhelmed, try general anti-anxiety affirmations.

♦ *I have more than enough time to get everything done. I am calm, I am peaceful.*

♦ *Things work out for me. All is well. Today is a wonderful day.*

When I was experiencing a particularly stressful time when my now-teenage children were a baby and a toddler, I would sing, "I am happy, I am strong, I am peaceful all day long." It served as a reminder that I could be. When we act as if we already are healthy, wealthy, and happy, we are halfway there. The common saying, "fake it 'til you make it" is the intent behind affirmations. You are telling yourself that something is already that way, and therefore your body responds by calming down.

When you make affirmations part of your daily life, everything flows with more ease and grace. The idea is that form follows thought. We manifest what we put our energy toward. Where thought goes, energy flows. Create your own affirmations, using your own words so they are meaningful for you.

Affirming that something is a certain way, such as "I am healthy and strong," is a form of positive thinking. I believe that on a cellular level the body hears the message and believes it. The repetition creates a belief in the body as well as the mind, and pretty soon, it is the truth. It also works in conjunction with our other behaviors. If we are trying to be healthier, repeating these affirmations will help reinforce healthy behaviors, such as eating nutritious food and exercising.

However, it must be said that *just* affirming will not make it so. We must put the steps in place to make the changes.

Studies are beginning to support affirmations. According to a 2013 study by J.D. Creswell, self-affirmation improves problem solving and performance on tasks related to executive functioning. Whether there is hard science backing affirmations or not, if they make us feel better and calmer, they are worth trying.

Action Item: Incorporate affirmations into your daily practices.

More reading: *You Can Heal your Life* by Louise Hay (Hay House Publishing, 1999)

Chapter 2

$\mathcal{B}$: Breathe

"For Breath is life, so if you breathe well you will live long on earth." Sanskrit proverb

Feeling stressed? Right now, take a deep breath. Inhale to a count of four. Pause for a count of one. Exhale to a count of eight. Repeat this type of breathing for about five minutes, and you'll feel calmer.

Breathe, inhale and exhale. Breathing is something we all do all day, every day. But we can actually manipulate our breathing to make it work more beneficially and efficiently.

Many people are chest breathers, holding the breath in the chest and making the breathing shallow, which means not using the full lung capacity. Shallow breathing causes nervousness, it doesn't fully oxygenate the blood, and therefore we have less energy.

If we take full, deep inhales and exhales, we give our bodies the gift of the breath. When we are feeling stressed and anxious, the simple act of taking one deep breath has the power to calm us down. It can slow a racing heartbeat and calm an agitated mind.

In his book *Autobiography of a Yogi*, Paramahansa Yogananda states that species that breathe more slowly live longer. He says that giant tortoises, which typically live upward of 150 years, take only four breaths per minute, compared with humans who take between twelve and twenty breaths per minute. If we take long, deep yogic breaths, our minds are calmer and less agitated, our bodies more relaxed. Conscious breathing may actually lengthen our lives.

Here are some breathing exercises to try.

Belly breathing: This simple breathing exercise can be done at any time. It is calming, relaxing, and can help get our bodies ready for sleep. Lie down on your back and place both hands on your belly, fingers toward the navel. Inhale to a count of four, allowing the belly to rise. Imagine a balloon in your mid-section slowly filling with air as you inhale. When the balloon is full, pause for a count of one and then exhale to a count of eight. As you exhale, imagine the air leaving the balloon. Do this exercise for five to fifteen minutes or until you either calm down or fall asleep, if you are using it as a sleep aid.

Ujjayi breath: This well-known yoga breathing technique can sometimes sound like the wind or a Darth Vader–type sound, but it doesn't need to. It is simply nose breathing with a partial constriction in the throat that slows the exhalation slightly. This type of breathing is done with traditional Ashtanga yoga, and the breath is directly correlated to the poses. For example, inhale while raising the arms to reach for the sky, exhale while folding forward. During a yoga practice, this type of breathing helps give the mind something to focus on, along with the gaze, or drishti. Benefits are a boost in energy and creating internal heat.

Alternate Nostril Breathing or Nadi Shodhana (channel purifying): The benefits of this technique include reduced anxiety and stress; lowered heart rate to relieve tension; revitalized mind and body; regulated cooling and warming cycles of the body; purified body channels so that energy, or prana, can flow more easily;

and prepared body for meditation. How to do it: Come to a comfortable seated position and sit tall, lengthening through the crown of the head. With your right hand, cover the right nostril with the thumb, and inhale slowly through the left nostril, then close the left nostril with the right ring finger. Remove the thumb from the right nostril, and exhale through the right nostril. Inhale through the right nostril, then close it with the thumb. Exhale through the left nostril, keep it open, then inhale through the left nostril. Cover with the ring finger, and exhale through the right nostril. Continue alternating like this for five to ten cycles. You may also rest the index and middle finger on the space between the eyebrows if that feels comfortable. Then relax with both hands resting in your lap and allow the breath to find its natural pace. This type of breathing can be done early in the morning or later in the day. It is also beneficial to practice Nadi Shodhana prior to meditation, as it calms us down by reducing anxiety.

Finally, here's a quick and easy breathing exercise for when you're feeling overwhelmed: Inhale to a count of four, hold the breath for a count of four, exhale to a count of eight. Repeat eight to ten times in a cycle to calm frazzled nerves.

In yoga, the breath is the bridge between mind, body, and spirit. It is through focusing on our breath that we begin to connect with spirit, to be present, to see what is really important. It helps take us out of our agitated monkey mind, a term used to describe the mind jumping from thought to thought like a monkey jumping from branch to branch. When we focus on the breath it calms us down. The best and quickest way to become centered is to take a deep, conscious breath.

The simple act of breathing in and breathing out with conscious awareness has the power to calm, to energize, to ground. When the world seems to be spinning out of control, just breathe. When it all seems too much to handle, just breathe. It may even extend your life.

Action Item: For more advanced breathing techniques, see a yoga teacher for pranayama exercises. See my website for videos.

More reading: *breathe, simple breathing techniques for a calmer, happier life*, by Jean Hall (Quadrille Publishing Ltd., 2016)

Chapter 3

C: Call a friend

"A good friend is a connection to life—a tie to the past, a road to the future, the key to sanity in a totally insane world." Lois Wyse

Call a friend. Connect. Talking to a friend, even if only for five minutes, can help ground us and make us feel better when we are feeling stressed. Women, especially, need to tend and befriend. It is part of our psychological make-up. When you are overwhelmed and you feel like you don't have five minutes to spare—find them! Call a friend and help yourself.

Research has long supported that a strong social network promotes physical as well as mental health. According to a review of 148 studies including 308,849 participants, people with stronger social ties had a 50 percent reduced risk of early death. This remained true independent of age, gender, initial health status, and cause of death.

People who lack social connections are more likely to experience elevated levels of stress and inflammation. These elevated cortisol levels can negatively impact the immune system and make the person more susceptible to immune issues and illness.

We are social beings, and our bodies function better when we are around other people. One of the main components to staying vital as we age is being around other people. In past generations, extended family members generally lived near or even with each other. In today's global world, young couples move away from their families of origin in search of career opportunities and adventure. When they have children, the new families are far from extended family and must find new support systems. Friends become the family substitute when family members are far away.

It is important for people to reach out to each other when they are feeling alone or experiencing stress and pressure. Because stress and pressure create a feeling of vulnerability, people with anxiety may retreat from social interaction, but this is when we most need connection. Checking in on our friends and neighbors will also help. We have no idea what people are going through unless we make the effort to find out.

It's beneficial to have friends in other age groups too. For example, everything changes in a woman's life when she has a baby. We sometimes feel as if we should instinctively and immediately know everything about raising a baby, but it is a steep learning curve—and scary to realize that it's up to us to keep this baby alive. Having a baby when far from family is a completely different experience than when people lived near extended family where other female family members—mother, grandmother, aunts, older sisters—could teach the new mother and watch the baby when the mother needed to rest.

Today, the mentor-type friend can help advise and reassure the young mother that what she is feeling and experiencing is normal. When you lack a built-in support system of family members, someone who's been there, done that, and who can offer wise and tested advice, is enormously beneficial. It's equally important for the new mom to have friends with kids around the same age, to compare notes about what is happening with her baby. For example, is it normal that they don't eat much initially and most of the food ends up on the tray or floor? Yes, it is!

One potentially tragic outcome of the social isolation new moms can feel is postpartum depression, which can become psychosis. Sometimes women cannot ask for the help they need and keep smiling on the outside while crying inside. In the worst scenario, they may harm themselves or their children.

It's important to have friends and stay connected through every stage of life, but the postpartum years are especially crucial. We tend to live isolated lives while seemingly being more connected than ever in our social media world. There are many helpful resources available online, but sometimes when you are in the thick of something you just need another human being to reassure you that everything is all right. And sometimes picking up the phone or meeting a friend for lunch or coffee is all we need. However, if you ever feel that you may harm yourself or your children, you need to seek professional help immediately.

National Suicide Prevention Lifeline:

1-800-273-8255

Action Item: If you are a new mom, join a playgroup or Mommy and Me music class so you have the opportunity to meet other moms with kids around your child's age.

More reading: *Down Came the Rain: My Journey through Postpartum Depression*, by Brooke Shields (Hachette Publishing, 2005)

Online: Check out mom of twin boys Michele Lovetri's blog In My Own Words at www.michelelovetri.com Instagram @michelelovetri

Chapter 4

D: Diet

"Food is fuel. Eat to live (don't live to eat)."
Anonymous

Improve your diet to include a wide variety of foods that provide nutrients for both brain and body health. We have all heard the phrase "you are what you eat." I believe there is truth to this saying. If we are jacked up on coffee and sugar, no wonder our hearts are racing, and we are bound to crash once the sugar high wears off. We can use what we eat to help us feel better, as there are many foods that help lower stress. Here is just a partial list of foods that help decrease anxiety levels.

- ♦ Leafy green vegetables contain folate, which helps the body produce dopamine, a pleasure-inducing chemical that helps keep us calm. In 2012, a study in the *Journal of Affective Disorders* found those who consumed the most folate had a lower risk of depression symptoms than those people who ate the least. Spinach, kale, collard greens, and broccoli are all high in folate.

♦ Blueberries and strawberries contain high levels of vitamin C and antioxidants, which fight free radicals that develop as a result of stress. These free radicals can weaken the immune system, and eating berries helps offset that stress response.

♦ Salmon contains omega-3 fatty acids with anti-inflammatory properties that may fight the negative effects of stress on our bodies. Omega-3s are also essential for optimal brain function and help prevent brain degeneration as we age. We can also get omega-3s from walnuts, flax seed oil, egg yolks, or a fish oil or flax seed oil supplement.

♦ Oatmeal has complex carbohydrates that can help the brain produce serotonin, a natural mood enhancer. Serotonin helps regulate anxiety and moods and helps increase feelings of happiness. Serotonin is like a natural antidepressant. While stress and the resulting cortisol release can cause a spike in blood sugar, a complex carb like oatmeal will help regulate it.

♦ Probiotic-rich foods like apple cider vinegar, kefir, some yogurts, kombucha, and sauerkraut help keep the gut healthy. Stress can cause problems in the intestines, which can then compromise the immune system and halt or slow production of the mood-boosting serotonin. Healthy intestine or gut flora is increased by eating probiotic-rich foods or by taking a high quality probiotic supplement.

♦ Nuts and seeds are good sources of magnesium. Studies show that magnesium helps reduce depression, fatigue, and irritability. Cashews, flax seeds, and pumpkin and sunflower seeds all have high magnesium levels and should be included in a healthy diet.

And now something to cut down on: caffeine. The headlines flip-flop from week to week as to whether caffeine consumption is beneficial or harmful, and I am not against coffee by any means. However, in my experience, I tend to be calmer when I am not drinking coffee. It sometimes makes my heart race and can make me jittery, particularly first thing in the morning and when I drink it on an empty stomach. If you have similar nervousness in the morning, I suggest trying a week without caffeine, just to see how you feel without it. Be aware that you may experience a withdrawal headache, but this will pass.

By implementing some of these changes into our diets, we improve our bodies' ability to handle stress and anxiety.

Action Item: Incorporate some of these stress-busting foods into your diet. Reduce caffeine consumption.

Chapter 5

E: Energy Healing

"Love is infectious and the greatest healing energy." Sri Baba

We are made of energy, which goes by many names including chi, ki, qi, and prana. Many types of hands-on healing can be helpful in balancing our chakras and keeping our etheric energy levels in good order before illness can manifest in the body. There are many different modalities to explore.

It makes sense that our energy can get depleted. One of the benefits of being trained in an energy healing modality is that you can and should give yourself treatments to keep your own energy flow strong and vibrant.

To picture the chakras—which travel along the meridians or energy pathways in Chinese medicine—

imagine seven spinning wheels of light along the spine, each a different color. They are red, orange, yellow, green, light blue, indigo, and violet. An energy worker clears those circuits so energy can flow freely from the giver to the receiver. The energy may be felt as heat, tingling, pulsing, or relaxation as it flows to specific places in the body/mind/spirit. Energy healing can be used regularly to balance the chakras, or when a person feels off center.

People tend to seek out energy healing treatments when they have a physical ailment and want to be healed. But energy healing works on all levels, starting with the aural or etheric levels. By the time something presents in the physical body, it has been around for a while. There is no guarantee that energy healing will cure someone, but an energy healing session will at the very least feel relaxing and often will bring the recipient pain relief. It is common for people to go into a meditative state while experiencing a treatment.

The best way to use energy treatments is as maintenance, so issues can be taken care of in the etheric energy levels; then they may never manifest in the body. It is just another way to take care of ourselves. Remember, too, that healing and curing are not the same thing. A person can experience deep healing and still not be cured of a disease or ailment. And sometimes an illness helps us learn or grow spiritually.

Energy healing also works on mental issues such as anxiety. It can calm us down and help alleviate stress and anxiety.

These are some types of energy healing to explore.

Therapeutic Touch: This is a contemporary interpretation of several ancient hands-on healing practices, developed by Delores Krieger PhD, RN, professor emeritus of Nursing at New York University; and Dora Kuns, an energy healer. Therapeutic Touch is categorized as a biofield energy therapy by the National

Center for Complementary and Integrative Health (NCCIH). NCCIH notes that although scientists are studying these techniques, not enough research currently exists to prove that they work. A typical session lasts about thirty minutes and consists of the practitioner centering themselves, assessing the client's energy field, clearing and balancing the client's energy field, evaluating and closing the treatment, and asking for feedback and answering client questions.

Reiki: The word *reiki* (pronounced ray-key) is used in Japan to mean any healing process that involves the use of the life force and is described as energy work. *Rei* means spiritual consciousness or divine wisdom that understands the person, their problems, the cause, and how to heal. *Ki* is the universal life force that animates all living things. It is the divine wisdom (or rei) that guides the life force (ki) in healing work. Therefore reiki is defined as spiritually guided life force energy. It cannot harm and can only help, as it is channeled through the light. It is an intelligent energy, going where it is needed. Even if the recipient does not consciously believe in God, the universe, the Source, or a universal power, reiki can still work. However, if at a soul level the recipient does not want help, it will bounce off and return to the sender. Sometimes people need to experience something for their own growth and will refuse help. Reiki is a safe, nurturing, noninvasive modality that does not drain energy from the practitioner, who is a conduit for the energy, as it comes from the Source. The reiki practice supports all other healing modalities. Reiki is also complementary to standard western medical and homeopathic treatments and is becoming more common in hospitals.

Quantum Touch: Similar to reiki and therapeutic touch, quantum touch is a hands-on modality that works with the recipient's energy field. Practitioners use breathing, body awareness, and hands-on techniques to focus and increase life-force energy. When this field of high energy is placed around an area of pain or inflammation, the body matches the higher energy frequency, creating an opportunity for self-healing. Quantum touch was created by Richard Gordon.

EFT: Emotional Freedom Technique, or tapping, is very simple to learn and is done by the individual simply tapping on certain parts of their body. It can provide relief from chronic pain, phobias, PTSD, addictions, disorders, and emotional and physical problems. Similar to acupuncture and acupressure, tapping is a set of techniques which use the body's energy meridians. You can stimulate these meridian points by tapping on them with your fingertips— tapping into the body's own energy and healing power. Tapping gives you the power to heal yourself.

Online: EFT: thetappingsolution.com; Quantum touch: quantumtouch.com; Reiki: www.reikialliance.com; Therapeutic touch: therapeutictouch.org

More Reading: *Reiki for Life*, by Penelope Quest (Penguin Group, 2002)

Chapter 6

$\mathcal{F}$: Forgiveness

"Through forgiveness, we create new realities that allow us to experience greater love and freedom." Iyanla Vanzant

Forgive yourself and others for past mistakes. That time is over. If we cling to old hurts, we are the ones who suffer. There are many different ways to forgive someone. If there is a memory or grievance that you've been holding on to, write a letter to the person or people involved. End the letter with forgiveness. After reading the letter, burn it in a metal bowl or pot. Bury the ashes, preferably in a garden or when you plant a new tree. That way you can symbolically use your past hurts to help something lovely grow.

Set yourself free, as well as the people who hurt you. Thank them for all they've taught you, and release the memories. See if this makes you feel lighter and freer. Not forgiving someone tends to hurt us far more than it hurts the person we need to forgive. They might not even be aware we are still holding on to pain from the past. Although we may not wish to, we all hurt each other at times; it is part of our learning journey on Earth.

There is a Hawaiian saying, "Ho'oponopono," which roughly translated means to make right again. It goes like this: I'm sorry, please forgive me, thank you, I love you. It is a catch-all that covers everything. If you have someone in mind whom you have hurt, close your eyes, lie down, and think about the person. Say their name in your mind, then say, I'm sorry, please forgive me, thank you, I love you. Repeat this, similar to saying a mantra, until you start to feel better. It doesn't matter if the person is still on Earth or has crossed over; it works, and on some level they will get the message. I have used this many times when memories of hurting someone come to mind. I believe we learn and grow throughout our lives, and when we know better, we do better. We are meant to make mistakes. We are not perfect. We are human.

Take out a sheet of paper and write, I forgive _____ for _____ _____. Repeat for three more people. Then repeat the exercise, forgiving yourself.

Doing this exercise will make you feel lighter, as if you've taken off a fifty-pound backpack. It is time to forgive yourself and others, so do it today!

Action Item: Practice Ho'oponopono whenever you feel the need to forgive someone.

More Reading: *ForGIVEness: 21 Days to Forgive Everyone for Everything* by Iyanla Vanzant (Hay House UK Limited, 2017)

Chapter 7

G: Go Outside/Ground

"Walk as if you are kissing the earth with your feet."
Thich Nhat Hahn

Spend time in nature. Studies show that the more time we spend outside, the happier and better able we are to deal with life's stressors. Try to go outside every day. In any season, our bodies benefit from fresh air and being in nature. Benefits of spending time outside include

- improvement in short-term memory. In one study from the University of Michigan, subjects were given a memory test, then divided into two groups. One group took a walk around an arboretum, and the other group walked down a city street. After the walk, they were tested a second time. The group that walked in the trees scored 20 percent higher than the original test score, while the group that walked in the city did not show an improvement over their original scores. In a second study, it was shown that among depressed people there is an increase in memory span after a walk in nature versus a city walk. For this study, twenty people diagnosed with MDD (Major Depressive Disorder) participated. The participants showed significant increases in memory span after the nature walk compared with the urban walk.

♦ increase in Vitamin D level. Vitamin D is necessary for maintaining a healthy immune system. A lack of vitamin D can increase chances of osteoporosis, cancer, and Alzheimer's disease. With the current focus on skin cancer, kids and adults often do not get enough vitamin D due to overapplication of sunscreen. Going out in the sun with no sunscreen early in the morning or later in the afternoon, when the sun isn't at its greatest strength, is the best time to get that daily dose of sunshine and vitamin D. Vitamin D also strengthens the bones, through calcium absorption, and helps regulate blood pressure, weight, and mood. Plus, it supports heart health as the heart contains many vitamin D receptors.

♦ improved mental health. According to researchers at Stanford University, people who walked for 90 minutes in nature as opposed to walking in an urban setting "showed decreased activity in a region of the brain associated with a key factor in depression," but the research reported little physiological differences for those who walked for 90 minutes in a city. Another Stanford study showed that subjects who walked in nature experienced less anxiety and more positive emotions than those who did not.

♦ improvement in academic performance. A study in Finland of boys and girls in first through third grades found that vigorous outdoor activity had a direct correlation to better reading comprehension and arithmetic skills, especially in boys. This doesn't surprise me at all. I am a mom of two boys, and boys definitely need to run it out and burn off excess energy in order to focus.

♦ lowered stress levels. David Strayer, a cognitive psychologist at the

University of Utah, has studied nature's calming effect on human stress levels. He was quoted in *National Geographic* as saying, "When we slow down, stop the busywork, and take in beautiful natural surroundings, not only do we feel restored, but our mental performance improves too."

"Grounding" or "earthing" are relatively new terms for going outside barefoot and literally connecting with the earth. Adults, especially, do not spend nearly enough time outdoors. Electronics constantly emit EMFs (Electromagnetic Frequencies), which can be harmful. One way to balance these harmful effects is by walking barefoot outside. Grounding balances the body's electrical energy with Earth's rhythms and can improve immune system health. Grounding also improves healing and recovery time by decreasing cortisol levels and reducing fatigue.

Think about how you feel when you are in a forest and cannot hear traffic sounds. It brings me back to when I was a child. There were lots of undeveloped wooded areas near my house, and my siblings and friends and I would explore them for hours.

There was a creek where we would catch crayfish, woods where we could climb trees and walk and explore. As more and more land is developed, there are fewer wooded areas. That, combined with "helicopter parenting" and overscheduling, means fewer kids have the opportunity to be free and explore the natural world.

Action Item: Walk barefoot on the grass, and see how it makes you feel. Walk barefoot around a labyrinth. Spend some time outside every day. If you live in a city, go to a park regularly to get your nature fix.

Chapter 8

$\mathcal{H}$: Help Someone Else

"I cried because I had no shoes until I met a man who had no feet." Persian saying

No matter what is happening in your life, helping others who have less, or need help more than you do, will keep you present and less likely to catastrophize your own issues. Many studies indicate that helping others increases our own happiness. But more importantly, helping others makes us feel good.

When researchers at the London School of Economics examined the connection between volunteering and measures of happiness in a large group of adults, they found a correlation between frequency of volunteering and happiness. Compared with people who had never volunteered, the odds of being very happy rose 7 percent among those who volunteer monthly and 12 percent for people who volunteer every two to four weeks. Among the weekly volunteers, 16 percent felt very happy.

When we help others, we get out of our own heads. I have volunteered in soup kitchens, and it is a serious reality check to come face to face with people who don't have enough money to eat, or who don't have a home. I was in high school the first time I helped at a soup kitchen, and I saw a boy around my age; I was sixteen at the time. I remember thinking, *this boy is just like me, he goes to high school, and yet he doesn't know where his next meal will come from.* It made me sad. I could tell he felt uncomfortable, too, from his body language. It was an eye-opening moment for my teenage self.

In my experience, anxiety tends to escalate. If we can feel it beginning, we can redirect our energy and then it subsides, or it can escalate into a full-blown panic attack. At that point, it is too late and we need help to calm down. The key is to put together processes so anxiety doesn't reach the level of a panic attack. When we help others, we begin to realize that we are not alone and that our problems and issues are not as terrible as we thought they were.

While the terms "champagne problems" and "first world problems" definitely resonate with me, the sensations that our bodies feel when being flooded with adrenaline from anxiety are no different than what our ancestors must have felt when they were battling each other or fleeing from a predator. Our bodies don't differentiate between a life-threatening situation and the stress of being late and stuck in traffic. The body reacts the same exact way whether the worry is self-created or a genuine fear for survival in the moment.

So help someone else, and help yourself. Look into volunteer programs in your area that interest you. It doesn't have to be a soup kitchen; you could volunteer to help an older person grocery shop, or go to a nursing home and visit patients who don't have family nearby, or become a big brother or big sister. The options are endless. One of my most rewarding teaching experiences was teaching seniors yoga at an assisted living community.

Action Item: Volunteer to help in whatever area you are passionate about. If you love reading, read to children at a local library. If animals are your thing, you can help at your local ASPCA.

Chapter 9

I: Indulge Yourself

"An empty lantern provides no light. Self-care is the fuel that allows your light to shine brightly."
Anonymous

Do something that pampers you, something you normally wouldn't do. Go to a spa and have a mud bath. Take an aerial yoga class. Have a manicure or pedicure. Better yet, do it with a friend. Then you can see your friend *and* take care of yourself. Caring for ourselves in this way may feel too self-indulgent, particularly if we're always caring for others. But it is equally as important to care for ourselves as it is to care for others. In fact, it is necessary. Caring for our appearance is not overly vain; it is part of taking care of our body, mind, and spirit.

I think of the body as a car, a high-performance vehicle that needs to be well maintained in order to run properly. It needs to have the best quality fuel (high quality food), it needs a weekly car wash (grooming), and it must have periodic oil changes and repairs and regular upkeep (doctor visits, preventative care) to keep it running at its optimal level. Self-care is essential for good health.

Here are some other ways to indulge yourself. They will take you out of your regular routine and make you feel pampered and special. You are special and should treat yourself as such.

- Get a hot stone massage.
- Go to a rock climbing gym.
- Get a haircut or blowout.
- Try something new, like a salt cave, ifloat water treatment, dance, or yoga on a paddleboard.
- Buy yourself flowers.

♦ Take a creative class such as painting, flower arranging, knitting, or photography—something you don't normally do.

♦ Go to a play or a show with a friend.

♦ Go on a girls' trip overnight.

More Reading: *The Art of Extreme Self-Care, Transform Your Life One Month at a Time*, by Cheryl Richardson (Hay House, 2009)

Action item: Schedule a weekend just for you at a spa or Kripalu, Omega, or Canyon Ranch.

Chapter 10

J: Journal

"Fill your paper with the breathings of your heart."
William Wordsworth

Writing things down helps us work through issues. Whenever I am feeling overwhelmed, I write down lists of what I need to do. Making journaling a habit helps keep thoughts from getting out of control.

Writing down feelings always helps. If I am experiencing something that causes me pain or sadness, sometimes I write a letter to the person who hurt me. It doesn't matter if I ever send the letter; it is more about getting my feelings out. Feelings of anger or sadness can get "stuck" in our bodies and cause pain, tightness, or even illness, which is why it is so important to talk about tough feelings such as anger or sadness. Writing them down is a way of dealing with them if we have trouble expressing them to the people directly involved, and that's where journaling comes in.

Buy yourself a pretty notebook and begin to write. Here are some journaling prompts:

> I am feeling anxious right now because . . .

> I can make myself feel better by . . .

> I am happy and calm when . . .

This type of journaling helps with expressing our feelings. We can also use journaling as a means to

- ♦ practice writing.
- ♦ organize thoughts or our to-do list for the day.
- ♦ keep track of ideas when we're out and about. I usually have a small notebook with me to jot down ideas as they come to mind. Ideas and thoughts can be fleeting and sometimes disappear if we don't write them down. I know we all carry phones

and could also record this in the notes section of the phone, but I just like the act of writing, pen to paper.

♦ find a creative outlet.

♦ keep track of dreams.

Action Item: Get a notebook and start a journal today.

Chapter 11

$\mathcal{K}$: Kick Toxic People Out of Your Inner

Circle

"Toxic relationships not only make us unhappy, they corrupt our attitudes and dispositions in ways that undermine healthier relationships and prevent us from realizing how much better things can be." Michael Josephson, ethics expert

You may be obliged to see people who tax you mentally or emotionally because you come in contact with them through work or because they are family members, but you can choose who you let become close to you.

You can always protect yourself by creating an energy barrier that only lets positive energy out and in. Here's how to do it.

Stand with your feet hip-width apart and place your hands on your heart. Intend in your heart and say either aloud or in your mind, "I am placing a sphere of self-protection around myself. Only good will flow out and only good will flow in. Any bad or negative energy will simply bounce off the barrier." Fill this sphere with golden healing light.

You can also set boundaries and limit the time you spend with toxic people. If you must spend time with people who drain your energy, here is an exercise to cut their emotional drain on you.

There are invisible psychic energy cords running between us and those with whom we are connected emotionally. This is why we sometimes know or sense when something is happening with that other person. With positive, loving relationships, this is a good thing. With energy vampires, it's a negative scenario. The exercise is simple. After spending time with someone who you feel drains your energy, make a karate chopping motion around your body, as if cutting through the energetic cords. Intending "I am cutting ties with _____" is all you need to do.

If you feel like a friendship or relationship is lopsided, with you always giving and the other person always taking, it is time for a conversation about boundaries. In the past, I have simply ended a friendship because I felt the other person was too negative. I used the excuse "it's not you, it's me," which was true. I was growing in a different direction and she did not fit in with my growth. I am ashamed now that I didn't have the courage to tell her the real reason. I might have been able to help her change had I been more specific as to why I was moving away from her, although in my experience, people change when they are ready to, and she probably wouldn't have accepted my opinion anyway.

Ways to deal with energy vampires:

♦ End the relationship.

- If this is not an option, limit time spent with this person.
- Try to only see this person when in a group and not alone.
- Protect yourself with an energy barrier.
- After spending time together, cut the emotional/energetic cords.

More Reading: *Emotional Vampires* by Albert J. Bernstein, PhD (McGraw–Hill Education, 2012). *Dodging Energy Vampires: An Empath's Guide to Evading Relationships that Drain You and Restoring Your Health and Power* by Dr. Christiane Northrup (Hay House Inc., 2018)

Chapter 12

L: Love

"Let yourself be silently drawn by the strange pull of what you really love. It will not lead you astray." Rumi

Let love be the driving force behind everything you do. Whenever possible, follow your bliss. Of course, we all need to do things that aren't our favorite things, but whenever possible we should choose love. For example, if we are doing the dishes or cleaning the house or something that is decidedly not blissful, we can put on happy music and dance while dusting.

Build pockets of peace into your day and whenever you can, choose love. If you need to drive your kids to practice and sit in the car to wait for them, bring an uplifting book to read while you wait.

Self-love is the most important type of love to master. When we love ourselves, we take care of ourselves and don't tolerate bad behavior. When we love ourselves, we can enter into a loving relationship knowing we are already whole and we don't need the other person, we simply want them in our life to enhance it.

You can practice being loving in relationships too. I believe that in all relationships there are moments when we feel less than loving, for whatever reason. But we can choose to love. Even if I do not feel loving, I can hug my partner or child or friend. We might be annoyed, but we can override the feelings of annoyance by letting go of the negative emotion and choosing to love instead.

When we are angry, sad, or stuck, it's important to feel the emotion, get it out, and then follow your joy. We don't want to suppress emotions or they can get stuck in our bodies, causing tension or even illness. Tension is just stress and unexpressed emotions blocking the energy pathways, so it is important to feel emotions and then release them. For example, if something happens and it's inappropriate to cry where you are, you can excuse yourself and quietly cry in a restroom. But the emotion needs to be expressed. After expressing it, try to do things to shift the negative mood to a positive mood. It seems simple because it *is* simple. It is not complicated to find ways to lead a happier, more fulfilling life.

Action Item: Follow your bliss. Do what brings you joy.

Chapter 13

$\mathcal{M}$: Music

"Where words fail, music speaks." Hans Christian Andersen

Feeling overwhelmed? Play a song that makes you want to sing out loud. Music lifts us up. Music brings us joy. Play whatever type of music you love, whenever and as often as you can. If you are prone to anxiety and depression, which often go hand in hand, using music to lift your spirits can help tame the anxiety before it takes over. Pop music usually makes me happy, but sometimes show tunes do the trick, and sometimes I need a song from childhood or adolescence to sing and dance to.

Research has supported that music, particularly classical music, can reduce blood pressure, slow heart rate, and provide other benefits for our autonomic nervous systems. Classical music not your jam? Not to worry, research also supports other types of music having similar benefits.

A 2013 study at McGill University in Quebec, conducted by Professor Daniel J. Levitin, reviewed more than four hundred research papers about the neurochemistry of music as it affected patients' stress prior to surgery. They found that listening to music helped reduce patient anxiety and also improved immune function. The music prescription was as effective or more effective than prescription medication in reducing patient anxiety.

The following are benefits of music to psychological well-being, according to research studies.

- ◆ The form and structure of music can improve the quality of life of distressed and disabled children by bringing order and security to their lives.

- Hospital patients awaiting surgery have lower stress levels while listening to music through headphones.

- Music can help lessen the severity and sensation of pain in hospital patients with chronic pain and postoperative pain.

- Listening to music can reduce feelings of depression and increase self-esteem ratings in elderly people.

- Music therapy significantly boosts quality of life among adult cancer patients by reducing feelings of depression.

Music has long been considered one of the great creative contributions to society, but now it is gaining credibility as a healing art as well.

Action Item: Go see a live band or orchestra performance.

More reading: *This is Your Brain on Music*, by Daniel J. Levitin (Plume/Penguin, 2007)

Chapter 14

$\mathcal{N}$: Now!

"Be here now." Baba Ram Dass, spiritual visionary

Look around and really be here. Give your full attention to the person you are with. Try really paying attention to what you're doing. Being mindful and giving mundane tasks our attention helps reduce stress.

Washing Dishes Exercise (Buddhist)

Take your time washing the dishes. Really pay attention to every sensation. Notice your senses.

Sight: Look at what you are doing. Be in the moment. See all the details of the dish. What color is it? Is it a round plate or a bowl or a frying pan?

Touch: How does it feel? Is it smooth, textured, heavy or light in your hand? Is it fragile, like crystal or china?

Do you need to be careful with it? How does the water feel? Is it hot?

Smell: What are the smells? Can you smell the residue of food and is it unpleasant? Do you enjoy the smell of the dish detergent? How do the scents make you feel?

Hearing: Does the sound of the rushing water drown out other sounds so you can really get lost in the moment? Is it a calming background noise? Is it jarring or disturbing to you if pots hit one another or a dish slips out of your hand?

Noticing what is happening as we go about our daily tasks helps keep us engaged and helps calm us down.

Mindfulness has been proven to reduce anxiety and depression. When we are present in the moment, we cannot regret the past or worry about the future. When we are present, we are right here, right now. Decisions and action happen in the present moment, and life is made up of a series of present moments, connected by our breath.

After many recent school shootings, I was very worried about my boys going to school, as I'm sure many people were. After 9/11, air travel changed forever. If we allow anxiety about what might happen rule our actions, we may never leave our houses. Being present and practicing mindfulness helps us stay focused on what is actually happening here and now.

Worry is wasted energy. Being present now, in each moment, we realize that everything is fine, until it may not be. But to worry about something that may never come to pass only drains our own energy and steals the joy from our lives. If we are worrying what *if*, we miss what *is*. We miss our life that is happening right now.

Mindfulness can help reduce stress. According to a study on present moment awareness, mindfulness has been shown to increase an adaptive response to daily stressors. Another study by Donald and Atkins (2016) showed that mindfulness produced less avoidance and more coping than relaxation or self-affirmation controls. My takeaway from these findings is that being present in each moment equips us to best handle issues when they arise.

Here are some tips to becoming more mindful each day.

- ♦ Stay focused on the task at hand.
- ♦ Notice everything as it comes into your experience.
- ♦ Acknowledge and accept the current situation.
- ♦ Stay grounded and make decisions from your center.
- ♦ Live with an open heart and mind.
- ♦ Be present, but also set goals for the future.

More Reading: *Wherever You Go, There You Are, Mindfulness Meditation in Everyday Life*, by Jon Kabat-Zinn (Reed Business Information, 1994)

Chapter 15

O: Optimist—Be One

"We can complain because rose bushes have thorns, or rejoice because thorn bushes have roses." Attributed to Abraham Lincoln

I don't believe we should have unrealistic expectations about life, but we should try to see the glass as half full. Looking on the bright side generally makes us happier. Things might be bad at any given moment, but they always improve. The sun will shine again after a rainy day, and that rain is needed to make the plants and trees grow. Maybe sometimes we need hard times to allow us to appreciate the good times.

I believe we are here to learn, to live our best lives, to love and to help each other. Not everyone is at the same level in their evolution. But this book is about increasing your own peace, and it is in *your* best interest to see things in a positive, rather than negative, light. If we believe we can do something, we are halfway there. If we believe we can't, we almost certainly won't; we beat ourselves before we even start.

Studies support the idea that optimists are healthier than pessimists. According to multiple United States and European studies, optimism helps improve health. Optimism helps patients cope with ailments and recover more quickly from surgery.

Optimists live longer. Research shows that an optimistic outlook early in life can predict better health and a lower rate of death during follow-up periods of fifteen to forty-plus years.

Scientists came up with two ways to measure optimism:

1. Dispositional optimism. This measures positive expectations for the future. These are generalized expectations for good outcomes in several areas of life. Researchers use a 12 Item Life Orientation test to measure these outcomes.

2. Explanatory style. This is based on how a person explains good or bad news. The pessimist assumes blame for bad news (it's me, it's all my fault), believes the situation is permanent (it will last forever), and has a global impact (it will affect everything I do). In contrast, the optimist takes credit for good news, expects that good things will last, and feels confident that positive outcomes will expand into other areas of their life.

According to two studies, one from the United States and one from the Netherlands, optimism improves overall health and therefore longevity. One study, beginning in the 1960s, looked at 6,959 students entering the University of North Carolina. The study included personality testing that rated students as either optimists or pessimists. It followed the students for forty years, during which time 476 participants died. Cancer was the most common cause of death, and the pessimists had a 42 percent higher rate of death during that period than the optimists.

The Dutch study reported similar results, evaluating 941 people between the ages of sixty-five and eighty-five. The subjects who demonstrated dispositional optimism at the study's beginning had a 45 percent lower risk of dying during the following nine years.

More Reading: *Learned Optimism* by Martin E. P. Seligman, PhD (Random House, 1991)

Chapter 16

$\mathcal{P}$: Play!

"Wanna come out and play?" All kids everywhere

Grab your kids or borrow someone else's. Run around outside or roll down a hill. Be childlike. Some of my best times are spent playing with my boys. We used to jump on the trampoline together or play basketball or wiffle ball. We usually ended up dissolving in laughter. Sometimes we still play, but now that they're teenagers they have less time and less interest in hanging out with their dad and me, which I totally understand.

Adults need time for play, just like children do. According to Dr. Stuart Brown, head of the National Institute for Play, adults use play as a way to connect with others. In San Francisco's Promenade Park there is a gaming club called SF Games. This group was started more than twenty years ago by David Kaye. The members gather around small card tables playing German games with figurines. These games are similar to American board games such as Monopoly, but they are inclusive, meaning people can play continually and not get excluded from the game.

Not only do adults not play enough, they don't laugh enough either. Children laugh an average of three hundred times per day, versus fifteen times per day for the average adult. Very happy adults may laugh one hundred times per day, according to Stanford professor William Fry. I decided to do an experiment to see how many times a day I laugh on average, which was about twenty times a day. I am trying to increase it. I am a happy person, generally speaking.

My fifteen-year-old son recently asked me what I do for fun. I had to really think about that. Exercise is fun for me, both teaching and taking classes. And I enjoy dancing and singing but rarely do those things. Why do we stop having fun as we get older? I love Disney movies, and one of the great joys of having kids was having a reason to go watch kid-friendly movies. Find what makes you feel like a kid again, and do that. There is no reason we should stop playing and having fun because we are adults. There is no reason we must lose our childlike wonder and sense of fun.

As a kid in Pennsylvania, I had morning and afternoon recess. In Connecticut they now have only one short break at lunchtime. Studies show that recess is declining in the United States, and currently only 16 percent of states have a mandate that elementary schools must provide recess for elementary school students, according to the *2016 Shape of the Nation* report. As time for standardized testing increases, time for recess decreases. The good news is that parents are fighting back and a few states (including Connecticut) have mandated that students must have twenty minutes of recess each day.

My family was fortunate to spend three years living in Australia where they have a much healthier balance between class and recess than we do in the United

States. Compared with our elementary school kids having barely twenty minutes of outside time each day, in Australia they were out for thirty minutes in the morning and an hour for lunch, for a total of ninety minutes every day.

This one goes for adults as well as kids. Why do many of us stop having fun when we grow up?

Action Item: Weather permitting, play Frisbee or fly a kite. If you live near the coast, go to the beach and build a sandcastle.

Chapter 17

Q: Quiet Meditation

"Quiet the mind and the soul will speak." Ma Jaya Bhagavati

Meditation can be as simple as sitting quietly, watching your breath for five minutes before starting your day. Find a comfortable position, close your eyes, and connect. This simple habit will put you in a great frame of mind for whatever the day brings. Taking five to fifteen minutes to be still and connect with your breath in the morning will give you increased energy and productivity throughout the day, even if you are busy. I had a friend tell me recently that she'd tried to meditate and "it's hard work." It doesn't have to be difficult. There are many different paths to meditation, from simply watching the breath and focusing on it, to guided meditation, to moving meditation, to transcendental meditation, which has its own set of rules and norms. It can be as simple or as complex as you need it to be. There are many courses and books to explore to find the right meditation for you.

Below, I give you some to try.

Morning Meditation

Here is an easy practice to begin your day strong and clear. Imagine that a giant ball of light, like the sun, is traveling around your body. Visualize this light filling any spaces of hurt, trauma, sadness, or pain in or around your physical, mental, or energy body. Feel the light filling and surrounding your body, removing any pain or sadness. Breathe deeply and sit with this feeling for five to ten minutes or longer if you have more time. When you come back, make sure to ground your feet and drink lots of water.

I believe we are all spiritual beings living in a human body while we are on Earth. We need to take the time to connect with our spiritual higher wisdom, because our spirit self or soul has greater knowledge than our human self does. We always have all the information, on a subconscious level, but when we agree to come to Earth, we make a deal that we will have amnesia for our time on Earth. We can't see the bigger picture because we are in Earth school, to learn by having a human experience. We are divine beings already, and our path on this planet is to remember our divinity and embody it fully, as we are destined to do. If you are at a crossroads in your life and seeking direction, this is the meditation for you.

Doors Meditation

Sit or lie down in a comfortable position and close your eyes. Begin breathing slowly and deeply. Allow your body to relax, and just focus on the breath for a few minutes. Notice how it feels when it enters your nose, as your belly rises and falls. Just get into a comfortable rhythm of following the breath.

Now visualize a house in front of you. Notice what color it is, how large; notice all the details. Walk up to the house and open the front door. Walk inside and look around. Notice the details of the room you are in, its color, its size. You will see a hallway to your right. Walk down the hallway. At the end of the hallway is a door. Open the door and go into the room. Notice the décor of the room. You will see a table with a chair in front of it. Have a seat at the chair. On the table is a small box. Open it. In the box is a piece of paper with a message on it. Take the piece of paper and read it. This is for you. The message on the piece of paper is meant for you, and it should have some meaning. If there is no message, do not despair; it will probably show up in a day or two. Sometimes we have to try a meditation multiple times before we get a message.

Wave Meditation

Sit or lie down in a comfortable position and close your eyes. Begin breathing slowly and deeply. Allow your body to relax, and just focus on the breath for a few minutes. Notice how it feels when it enters your nose, as your belly rises and falls. Just get into a comfortable rhythm of following the breath.

Imagine that you are floating on the ocean. A presence rises from deep within you and propels you forward. The wave is you, and you are the wave. The water is always changing shape as it moves within you. With each rising of the wave, you are created anew. The more you surrender to the power of the ocean within, the more you are moved effortlessly toward your destination.

As you inhale, feel the wave of love arise from within. As you exhale, imagine yourself floating and supported by an ocean of love. Keep breathing and feeling the water move through and inside you. Stay here for five to ten minutes or longer if you have more time.

When you bring yourself back from your meditation, you should feel relaxed and refreshed and ready to continue your day with lots of energy, but remember to stay hydrated and take your time grounding.

Action Item: Try the online Apps Calm and Headspace.

My website, www.LeaGrimaldi.com, has several articles and video meditations to explore.

Chapter 18

R: Reduce Clutter

"Clear clutter—make space for you." Magdelena Vandenberg

I believe we all have clutter thresholds beyond which we cannot take it anymore. Mine is definitely higher than my husband's. While it drives him crazy if the Tupperware cabinet is in disarray, it doesn't bother me a bit—I can always find the lid to match the container. However, I do admit that it is nice when everything is in order, and so I have been working on improving my organizational skills. I recently cleaned out my entire closet, which had been extremely disorganized. I gave a lot of stuff to Goodwill, the Veterans Association, and the Boys and Girls Club and it felt so freeing. I cleared out space and helped other people by donating stuff I didn't need any longer to people who could use it. Reducing clutter makes us feel physically and energetically lighter. It creates space. Extra stuff weighs on us and saps our energy.

My sister Kim told me about the donation closet at her workplace. The adage "one person's trash is another's treasure" applies here. Any employee can place items in the "magic closet" for someone else to use. The items disappear like magic. Kim checks it from time to time and recently found a great mixing bowl that was just the size she needed.

According to feng shui principles, when we clear clutter we remove blocks to our success. Piles of stuff in disarray actually can sap our energy so we have less energy to devote to what we want.

We can do a little bit every day to clear out our personal spaces. Here are some tips:

♦ Have a designated mail spot. Whether it is a folder on a counter, a place in a drawer, or a desktop basket, find a place for the mail to go. This way, important mail will not get misplaced, and you will have a spot to sort it.

◆ Have a place to hang your keys. I have a hook where I place my keys when I come home. This helps eliminate the stress of searching for the keys when it's time to leave the house, which is especially important for busy moms with many things to remember in the morning.

◆ When you come home, always hang up coats and put shoes away, and teach your kids to do the same.

◆ Every day, devote some time to cleaning up and clearing out. I learned this trick from my very wise husband: If you see something that needs to be done, do it. For example, while cooking dinner, if I notice that the refrigerator needs a wipe down, I can make use of my downtime (waiting for water to boil) by cleaning it. Make these mini cleanups part of your routine and your living space will always be in decent order.

Action Item: Do a spring/fall clean up every year and donate clothes and items you aren't using.

Chapter 19

S: Smile

"We shall never know all the good a smile can do. Start with a smile, for the smile is the beginning of love." Mother Teresa

Smile all the time, at everyone you see. When you smile, your body physiologically gets the message that you are happy. When you frown, it gets the message that you're sad. Your body doesn't know the difference between a real or a fake smile, so smile away!

According to a study by psychologists Tara Kraft and Sara Pressman, the body responds to a real smile or a fake smile by beginning a positive feedback loop where a message is sent to the brain that causes the release of endorphins—the happy brain chemicals—and thus makes you feel happier.

Their experiment had 169 participants hold chopsticks in their mouths in three different positions. A neutral face, a smile with the mouth only, or a Duchenne smile (a wide smile that engages the eyes as well). Only half of the participants were instructed to smile. Then the researchers had the subjects do a variety of stress-inducing tasks, such as tracing a star with their non-dominant hand while looking at a reflection of the star in the mirror. The researchers monitored their heart rates and self-reported stress level after completing the tasks. The results showed that the subjects who were instructed to smile had the lowest heart rate and reported less stress than those with the neutral expression. But even the subjects who were not specifically instructed to smile but had their faces forced into a smile by holding the chopsticks had lower stress and heart rates than the subjects with the neutral expressions.

Try it yourself. Next time you are stuck in traffic or experiencing some other type of stress, try holding your mouth in a smile and see if it makes you feel better. It might even lower your blood pressure and help your heart as well. If I am on the phone with a customer service representative and things are not going as planned and I am feeling frustrated, I will sometimes smile, and it does make me feel better. Try it!

Another study's findings support that smiling helps relieve depression. A study by cosmetic dermatologist Eric Finzi and Norman Rosenthal (Director of Psychology at Georgetown University) looked at the effect of facial expression on depressed patients. In their study were seventy-four subjects diagnosed with major depression. Some of the subjects were injected with Botox between the eyebrows, which prevented them from frowning. The others were injected with a placebo saline solution that had no effect. Six weeks after the injection, 52 percent of the non-frowning Botox group reported a reduction in their depression, compared with 15 percent of the placebo group. The results indicate that faking a smile really can make people feel happier.

It takes fewer muscles and creates fewer wrinkles for you to smile than to frown. We are social beings, and smiling shares our joy and love with others. In a world that is sometimes crazy, scary, and confusing, why not smile and spread joy?

In addition, people who smile more are perceived as being friendlier, happier, and nicer to be around than their nonsmiling counterparts.

Smiling reduces the stress that our bodies and minds feel, similar to getting enough sleep, according to recent studies. This explains why we feel happier around children—on average they smile four hundred times a day. Happy adults tend to smile forty to fifty times a day, while the average adult smiles just twenty times a day.

Years ago, while I was living in the West Village of New York City, I put some money in a homeless man's jar and smiled at him. In return he gave me a huge smile back, and said, "Thank you, especially for the smile. It makes me feel like a human being." More than twenty years later, that memory stays with me, as it illustrates the power a smile can have.

Smiling is definitely more than just a contraction of the facial muscles. In fact, Mother Teresa's quote was right on target!

Action Item: Smile at strangers.

Chapter 20

$\mathcal{T}$: Thank you! Say It Every Day

"If the only prayer you ever say in your entire life is thank you, it will be enough." Meister Eckhart

Do you feel stressed out right now? Write down three things that make you feel grateful. Feel better?

Begin a gratitude journal. The more we are thankful for, the more the universe rewards us. Writing a gratitude journal can be as simple as keeping a notebook near your bed. Each night, before going to sleep, write the date and three things for which you are thankful. They can be big or little things, it doesn't matter. The important thing is that you write them down and allow yourself to feel that gratitude. Being thankful attracts more good things to us. I am thankful for all the experiences in my life, even the ones that could be perceived as negative.

Every experience is a learning opportunity that brings us to today, and the people we are today. I started a Facebook Gratitude journal in 2017 and made it to day 101. Like everything, it is a practice. I started another one for 2019, and my plan was to have one entry for every day of the year. I have missed a few days but will make it to at least 350 this year. Since starting the journal, I feel calmer and happier. When we take the time to feel gratitude for what we do have, we are less stressed and more present. We are able to enjoy life more.

I often thank my body for all it does for me, every day. If we are struggling with losing weight or aren't happy with our appearance, we need to love our bodies where we are now, before we are able to change our habits and improve our health.

Psychology research supports this, as gratitude is consistently associated with greater happiness. In one study, two psychologists, Dr. Robert A. Emmons at the University of California, Davis, and Dr. Michael E.

McCullough at the University of Florida, asked participants to write down two sentences each week focusing on specific subjects. The first group wrote down what they were grateful for during the week, the second wrote about daily irritations, and the third wrote about something that happened but did not give it a positive or negative slant. After ten weeks, the people who wrote about gratitude were more optimistic and felt better about their lives. They also exercised more and had fewer doctor visits than the group that wrote about daily annoyances.

More reading: *The Gratitude Diaries* by Janice Kaplan (Harper Collins, 2017)

Action item: Start your own gratitude journal, either online or in a paper journal.

Chapter 21

$\mathcal{U}$: Unplug!

"Almost everything will work again if you unplug it for a few minutes, including you." Anne Lamott

No computer, iPhone, iPad, TV, anything electronic for a day or a weekend. Maybe have the whole family do it too, or your housemates. Notice how it changes your communication with each other. Notice how much time you have for other pursuits when you aren't checking your email, Facebook, Twitter, or Instagram every few minutes.

When we lost power for several days following Hurricane Sandy, we played Monopoly. We played cards. We went hiking. My boys were twelve and fourteen at the time, and extremely focused on their electronics. The devices ruled their thoughts. But for those few days, we really had great quality time together as a family.

I am going to do it again. They will probably fight me tooth and nail, but I know we'll all learn something from the experience. Everyone is constantly on their phones. It can't be good. Instead of stepping in to break up fights, kids record them and repost to try to get views. People can have hundreds or even thousands of "friends" on Facebook or Instagram, but how many of these people do they spend time with face to face on a regular basis?

Another way to unplug is to take a break from watching the news. I find when I avoid the news I am happier and calmer. I listen to NPR in the car, so I have a general working knowledge of what's happening, and of course I will turn the news on if I hear of a big news story. However, on a daily basis, watching the news just stresses me out. Research supports me on this one as well. According to a survey by the American Psychological Association, more than half of

Americans say watching or reading the news causes them stress, and many report feeling anxiety, fatigue, or sleep loss as a result of news consumption. (However, many of the survey respondents report checking the news feed on their phone or computer once an hour, with as many as 20 percent checking their social media feeds constantly, which includes the news headlines.)

Additionally, the way and format in which the news is delivered has changed drastically since the Web and smartphones came into existence, becoming more immediate and more shocking and personal. This bystander-captured media can cause acute stress, according to Graham Davey, editor-in-chief of the *Journal of Experimental Psychopathology* and professor emeritus at the University of Sussex University in the UK, and quoted in Time Online. "The way that news is presented and the way we access news has changed drastically over the last 15 to 20 years." With everyone holding a smartphone, bystanders will take videos that may end up on the nightly news. This adds to the stress and immediacy of news coverage. "These changes have often been detrimental to general mental health," said Davey.

Going on a news diet sounds like a good idea!

Action Item: Unplug for a weekend or week. Start phone-free mealtimes if the kids (or you) never put the phone down.

More Reading: *iGen* by Jean M. Twenge, PhD (Simon & Schuster, 2017)

Chapter 22

$\mathcal{V}$: Vacation

"A vacation is having nothing to do and all day to do it in." Robert Orben

Or as they say in Australia, holiday. Take one! It doesn't need to be a week-long trip involving a plane ride. It could be a weekend away. Or even just a Sunday drive to a new restaurant for lunch. This past summer, my husband and I had to travel to a town about forty minutes away for our son's baseball game, and we went out to lunch, which we rarely do. It was a nice, relaxing change of pace. We walked down a lovely main street and browsed in an antique store prior to the game starting, and it really felt like we had taken a vacation.

We are very fortunate to live near a beach, which we don't frequent nearly enough. This past summer, we went on a few weekend mornings and it was wonderful. It doesn't have to be a whole day trip—it can be an hour to recharge, dip your toes in the water, sit on the sand, and watch the seagulls. When we remove ourselves from our usual day-to-day surroundings, we return refreshed and full of peace and energy. And it doesn't have to be a beach. Anywhere away from your regular surroundings will work.

We were blessed to live in the suburbs of Melbourne, Australia for three years from 2008–2011. The Australian people really know how to live. They work to live, unlike living to work. They take long holidays. Part of the reason for this is probably because they are so secluded, and the jet-lag factor makes it almost not worth it to go anywhere for less than two weeks, and preferably more than two weeks. But part of it is just their culture.

Where we lived, in Brighton, Victoria, the town basically closed for the week between Christmas and New Year's Day. I remember I went to take my husband's clothes to the dry cleaner, and it was closed—all week. Local coffee shop, closed—all week. Produce grocer, closed—all week. You get the picture. They want to enjoy life, so they take long vacations and enjoy their holidays.

One year, we visited Sydney for New Year's Eve. Many restaurants and nightclubs were closed there for the week as well, during one of their busiest times of the year for tourism. It is summer in December there, and many tourists travel to Sydney to see the New Year's Eve fireworks. The Australians don't care. They will take time off at the risk of losing money, because their time and peace of mind is more important to them than money. It's a viewpoint that we in the United States could do well to adopt.

Action Item: Plan a vacation. Even just thinking about where we'd like to go relieves stress.

Chapter 23

W: Water

"I think I was a mermaid in another life." Anonymous

Water helps with stress relief in many ways, from staying hydrated to participating in water sports to sitting on a beach gazing at the ocean.

Drink up. Stay hydrated for stress relief. Even being slightly dehydrated can increase anxiety. Water plays a huge role in our physical processes, and when we don't have enough, cortisol levels rise. Cortisol is a hormone that makes us feel stressed and anxious. Water also plays a part in balancing mood, so staying hydrated means we are less likely to experience depression and anxiety. When the body is not properly fed and hydrated, it starts to produce more cortisol and adrenaline, to fuel its needs. This further triggers the stress response, and the cycle continues.

The amount of water each person needs varies depending on size, age, and activity level, but the Mayo Clinic advises drinking eight to ten eight-ounce glasses of water each day, or about 64 ounces. In stressful situations, it is important to drink even more water. If you are feeling anxious or stressed, a simple glass of water could bring your stress levels down. Adding caffeine to the mix of cortisol and adrenaline helps boost energy, but caffeine can also increase the release of cortisol. So if you do have coffee, make sure to drink one glass of water for each cup of coffee consumed.

Another way water helps us destress is simply its meditative quality. Whether an ocean, river, lake, stream, or pond, find a body of water and watch it. Feel your stress dissolve. Our bodies are made up of more than 60 percent water, and when we sit by water, we automatically feel better. Research suggests that walking or sitting near water signals the brain to release the happy chemicals, such as dopamine, for a natural high. Studies also support that surfing and enjoying the water can help veterans work through PTSD symptoms.

Since ancient times, rituals and gatherings have happened near the water, and today we often have weddings, celebrations, and vacations near or at an ocean, bay, or lake. It seems that we are programmed to feel good around water. According to marine biologist Wallace J. Nichols, we are. Something in our brains attracts us to it. He writes, "We are beginning to learn that our brains are hardwired to react positively to water and that being near it can calm and connect us, increase innovation and insight, and even heal what's broken."

Here are some of the main ways the brain benefits while we are near water.

> ◆ Water can induce a meditative state of mind. Many people enjoy sitting by the water and watching it. It can create a state of calm focus, somewhat similar to a meditative state. Being mindful can lower stress levels, relieve mild anxiety, reduce

pain and depression, and improve focus and sleep quality.

♦ According to research, people can experience feelings of awe when around water, which inspires a connection to something bigger than oneself. This may be why so many weddings are held near bodies of water, besides the photo op.

♦ Water helps get creativity flowing. I get many ideas in the shower, and I'd guess I'm not alone in this. In our busy, screen-dominated lives, we don't give our minds much opportunity to rest and wander. According to Nichols, stepping into the shower is similar to going to the ocean, albeit on a smaller scale. "You step into the shower, and you remove a lot of the visual stimulation of your day. Editorially, it's the same thing—it's a steady stream of 'blue noise.' You're not hearing voices or processing ideas. It's like a mini-vacation."

♦ Exercise near water to get the double benefit of the exercise plus the calming and stress-relieving benefits of water. Find a river or lake and jog or ride your bike. It is immediately calming.

Action Item: Find some water near your home or work and try to visit it weekly, whether by jogging along a river or sitting on a beautiful beach.

More Reading: *Blue Mind: The Surprising Science that Shows How Being Near, In, On, or Under Water Can Make You Happier, Healthier, More Connected, and Better at What You Do* by Wallace J. Nichols (Back Bay Books, 2015)

Chapter 24

X: eXercise!

"Take care of your body. It's the only place you have to live." Jim Rohn

Move your body every day. It is proven that consistent, regular exercise is more beneficial to combatting depression than pharmaceuticals. Exercise increases the "feel good" chemicals and decreases the "feel bad" ones. Exercise *is* the fountain of youth. It keeps us strong and healthy, gives us more energy, and helps keep our immune systems strong. The key is that it has to work with our lifestyle. So if you do not like a gym setting, try a boutique fitness studio or a rock climbing gym, or run outside, play tennis, or swim.

I have a friend who swam competitively as a child and in high school. She recently got back to swimming as an adult, and it feels like coming home to her. It is nonimpact so it's soothing for the joints and bones, and it brings her joy. This is what it's all about—love and joy. We need to find an exercise that we love, so we want to do it. It needs to be a lifestyle change. It needs to become automatic, like brushing our teeth.

Human beings need to move. We are not meant to be sedentary, sitting in a desk chair every day for our whole lives. Although modern conveniences are a wonderful thing, too much convenience can work against us. According to the National Center for Health Statistics (NCHS), in 2015–2016, 39.8 percent (about 93.3 million) adults in the United States were obese. This is the most recent statistic available. Processed foods, fast foods, poor food choices, technology, and lack of movement all contribute to this epidemic. But they also all work together. If we change one thing, for example, start moving our bodies more, we naturally start to make healthier food choices.

Exercise is truly the magic pill for feeling good at any age. Running, walking, yoga, weight training, spinning, group exercise, barre, boot camp—it doesn't matter. Move your body. If it gets your heart pumping and builds lean muscle, it enhances cardiovascular and muscular health. As we age, we need to keep exercise a priority to stay strong into old age. Incorporating weight training into the program will help keep balance strong to prevent falls.

If you are into middle age and have not yet made exercise a regular part of your lifestyle, now is the time to start, because this is what will keep you strong and vibrant for the rest of your life. Excluding a structural issue like kyphosis or scoliosis, the forward leaning posture that many associate with growing older is not inevitable. This is not a natural function of aging, but it can happen if our core muscles are weak. If we stay strong through regular exercise and we practice good posture, there is no reason to hunch over into old age. Think about women who were once ballet dancers; they are graceful, lithe, strong, and supple, even as elderly women. This is possible for us all.

Action item: Try a different exercise class with a friend each week for a month, with the goal of picking one at the end of the month. Make sure to get your doctor's approval.

Chapter 25

Υ: Yoga

"The yoga postures and breath are tools to rebuild and transform ourselves. The goal is not to tie ourselves in knots—we're already tied in knots. The aim is to untie the knots in our heart. The aim is to unite with the ultimate, loving, and peaceful power of the universe." Max Strom, yoga teacher

There are so many types of yoga to choose from that every person can find one that works for them. Here are some:

Bikram Yoga. Love sweating and intense heat (like over 100 degrees)? Try Bikram Yoga. It is always the same, twenty-six set poses, each performed twice, once for ninety seconds and then again for sixty. It is great for a good sweat and to detox but is not for everyone. If you don't like heat, this is not the yoga for you. It is a full ninety-minute class, which is a long time for a class, and because the room is so hot, unless you do not sweat at all you will sweat and therefore need to shower. Pros: cleansing, always the same, you can measure your progress, always feel lighter afterward. Cons: no music, bright lights, austere environment.

Ashtanga Yoga. True ashtanga is always the same, following a certain set of poses done in a specific order. There are DVDs that offer Ashtanga; a great one is by Beryl Bender Birch who wrote *Power Yoga* and was one of the first yogis to bring true Ashtanga to the United States. This is a very strong, athletic style of yoga incorporating sun salutations between every pose in the first series, which is a lot of vinyasas.

Vinyasa/flow yoga/Power Yoga. The true definition of *vinyasa* is poses linked together with the breath (as in plank, chatturanga, updog, downdog), but now many classes that are similar to Ashtanga are termed vinyasa or vinyasa flow. It is a flowing class rather than a class where poses are held for a longer time. Vinyasa flow teaches us to link the poses with the breath. It is a meditation in motion and also a strong physical workout.

Yoga Nidra/Yin Yoga. Yoga nidra means yoga sleep. This is generally a longer yoga class, an hour and a half to three hours long, including assisted deep stretching—long-held poses with bolsters and blankets for support. A deeply restorative practice, this is a wonderful add-on to your fitness repertoire, to let your body really stretch and relax.

If you are new to yoga, try a class and see what you think. Hatha yoga is a blanket term that means all types of physical yoga, but many studios use it interchangeably with gentle yoga. The important thing is to give it a try . . . and if going to a studio is not possible, you can rent a DVD at the library, buy one, or try a live-streaming yoga class.

Action Item: Try a local class or buy, rent, or borrow a DVD. "Baron Baptiste Introduction to Ashtanga Yoga" is a good place to start for Ashtanga. Bryan Kest's "Power Yoga" DVD series has three levels.

Chapter 26

Z: ZZZs–Catch Some

"Without enough sleep, we all become tall two-year-olds." JoJo Jensen

Sometimes our bodies just need a rest. Either a good, long nap or going to bed. Listen to your body and be sure to get enough sleep. Go to bed at the same time every night and try to get up around the same time in the morning. Of course everyone gets off track sometimes, but if we try to develop a sleep routine, we will be healthier and happier.

Busy is the new affliction. Too busy to spend time with friends, too busy to take care of ourselves, too busy to do what brings us joy. We must make the time to do the things that fill us up. We must make the time to be still. Our body, mind, and spirit cannot be on all the time, because we are not robots. We are human be-ings, not human do-ings. We need time to be quiet, to process. And with the ever-increasing technologies that bombard us every second of every day, it is even more imperative to take care of ourselves, rest, and unwind.

Results of sleep deprivation include

- depression.

- memory loss. During sleep, short-term memories are converted to long-term memories. Chronic sleep loss interrupts this important process.

- becoming accident prone. Insufficient sleep means we are more likely to make mistakes that can lead to accidents. For this reason, there are laws about how long truckers can drive without rest.

- weight gain. Insufficient sleep causes a spike in appetite. Being overtired during the day makes exercise more difficult, resulting in weight gain.

- increased mortality. According to a 2007 study in Great Britain, individuals who get just five hours of sleep per night double their chances of dying prematurely.

- loss of libido.

- aging appearance. When we aren't well rested, we don't look as good. Insufficient sleep causes cortisol, the stress hormone, to be released. Cortisol breaks down skin collagen, prematurely aging the skin.

- high blood pressure. A lack of sleep may lead to high blood pressure, which increases the possibility of a stroke.

- immune system weakening. A weakened immune system makes us more susceptible to illness.

- fatigue. While fatigue is an obvious side effect of sleeplessness, over time it can become chronic.

Sleep is a biological need, and insomnia feeds off itself and raises our anxiety. Think about the meltdowns toddlers have when they are overtired and haven't napped. It is the same for adults. When we aren't getting enough sleep, we cannot function as well as we can when we are sufficiently rested. It is fine to go without sleep for a certain amount of time, but when it becomes continual and prolonged, we cannot function properly and need to get help.

Here are some easy sleep strategies.

- ◆ Take a power nap, no longer than thirty minutes and you will wake up refreshed.
- ◆ Develop a regular routine of going to bed and getting up around the same time each day, so your body knows what's coming.
- ◆ Do not eat within an hour of bedtime. If your body is focusing on digestion, it won't be ready for a good night's rest.
- ◆ Try a melatonin supplement.

♦   If self-help measures aren't working, see a doctor for more assistance.

Get the rest you need, and your body will thank you.

Thank you for taking the time for yourself to read this book. It is my sincere hope that you have learned a technique—or three—to tuck into your toolbox, as these are all strategies that I use on a weekly (if not daily) basis. Please visit my website at LeaGrimaldi.com for meditation videos, my blog, and online courses. I am always available.

References

Berman, M. G., et al. "Interacting with Nature improves cognition and affect for individuals with depression." *J. Affect. Disord.* (November, 2012): 140(3): 300–5. doi:10.1016/j.jad.2012.03.012.

Berman, M. G., J. Jonides, S. Kaplan. (2008) "Going outside—even in the cold—improves memory, attention." *Psychological Science* (2008).

Borgonovi, F., (2008) "Doing well by doing good. The relationship between formal volunteering and self-reported health and happiness." *Social Science and Medicine*, 66, no. 11 (June 2008): 2321–2334. doi: 10.1016/j.socscimed.2008.01.011.

CDC. *National Health and Nutrition Examination Survey 2017.*

https://www.cdc.gov/nchs/data/factsheets/factsheet_nha nes.htm

Creswell J. D., J. M. Dutcher, W. P. Klein, P. R. Harris, J. M. Levine. (2013) "Self-Affirmation Improves Problem-Solving Under Stress." *PLoS ONE* 8, no. 5 (May 1, 2013): e62593. doi:10.1371/journal.pone.0062593.

Davey, G. C. L. "The psychological impact of negative TV news bulletins: The catastrophizing of personal worries." *British Journal of Psychology* 88, part 1 (February 1997): doi:10.1111/j.2044-8295. 1997.tb02622.

Donald, J. M., P. W. B. Atkins, (2016) Mindfulness and Coping with Stress: Do Levels of Perceived Stress Matter? *Mindfulness* 7 (2016): 1423–1436. doi:10.1007/s12671-016-0584-y.

Enqvist, I., J. Kulmala, J. Kallio, T. Tammelin. "Physical activity and sedentary behavior during outdoor learning and traditional indoor school days among Finnish primary school students." *Journal of*

Adventure Education and Outdoor Learning, 19, no. 1 (2018): 28–42. doi:10.1080/14729679.2018.1488594.

Finzi E., L. Kels, J. Axelowitz, B. Shaver, C. Eberlein, T. H. Krueger, M. A. Wollmer. "Botulinum toxin therapy of bipolar depression; A case series." *Journal of Psychiatric Research* 104 (September 2018): 55–57. doi:10.1016/j.jpsychires.2018.06.015.

Froh, J., W. J. Sefick, R. A. Emmons. "Counting blessings in early adolescents: An experimental study of gratitude and subjective well-being." *Journal of School Psychology* 46, no. 2 (2008): 213–233. doi:10.1016/j.jsp.2007.03.005.

Fry, W. F., "The physiologic effects of humor, mirth, and laughter." *JAMA* 267 (1992): 1857–1858. doi:10.1001/jama.267.13.1857.

Harvard Medical School. *Optimism and Your Health.* Harvard Health Publishing, May, 2008.

https:/www.health.harvard.edu/heart-health/optimism-and-your-health.

Holt-Lunstad, J., T. B. Smith, M. Baker, T. Harris, & D. Stephenson. (2015). "Loneliness and social isolation as risk factors for mortality: a meta-analytic review." *Perspectives on Psychological Science,* 10, no. 2 (March 2015): 227–237.

Kraft, T. L., S. D. Pressman. "Grin and bear it: the influence of manipulated facial expression on the stress response." *Psychological Science* 23, no. 11 (2012): 1372–8. doi:10.1177/0956797612445312.

Levitin, D. J., M. L. Chanda. "Music to treat pain and reduce stress." *Trends in Cognitive Sciences* (April 2013).

University of Warwick. "Short Sleep Increases Risk of Death & Over Long Sleep Can Indicate Serious Illness." *Sleep* (2010).

Yogananda, Paramahansa. *Autobiography of a Yogi.* (Los Angeles: Self-Realization Fellowship, reprint January 5, 1998).

About the Author

Lea Grimaldi is a yoga, barre, and meditation instructor with nineteen years' experience teaching yoga and fitness classes in health clubs, studios, and corporations to everyone from schoolchildren to athletes to an eighty-eight-year-old woman with two hip replacements.

Her education includes a BA degree from the University of Delaware in English with a Journalism concentration. Lea has worked in trade publishing for Miller Freeman, Inc. as an editor and writer. Lea has been a member of Yoga Alliance since 2008, E-RYT500, member of YTAA (Yoga Teachers Association of Australia) obtained while living Down Under. She is a practicing Reiki Master and offers reiki sessions under Yoga4U, her yoga and reiki business. She lives with her husband and two boys, her greatest teachers, in Connecticut. You can find her on Facebook at http://Lea.grimaldi.4/facebook.com and Instagram @lea_grimaldi

Acknowledgments

Thank you to my many clients and friends who have inspired this book, it has been a long time coming. Meredith Tennant, thank you for your expertise and suggestions. Thank you to my first readers; Nicola Mahoney, Lydia Elder, Cathleen Gelman, Becky Aurilio, April Guilbault, and Kim Segal-Morris. Your thoughtful comments helped to shape the final version, and I so appreciate your time. Finally, thank you to my best boys, husband Steve and sons Joel and Kyle, with whom everything is possible.